SUPER KETO DIET RECIPES

THE MOST DELICIOUS RECIPES TO LOSE WEIGHT QUICKLY

JACK HUDSON

Table of Contents

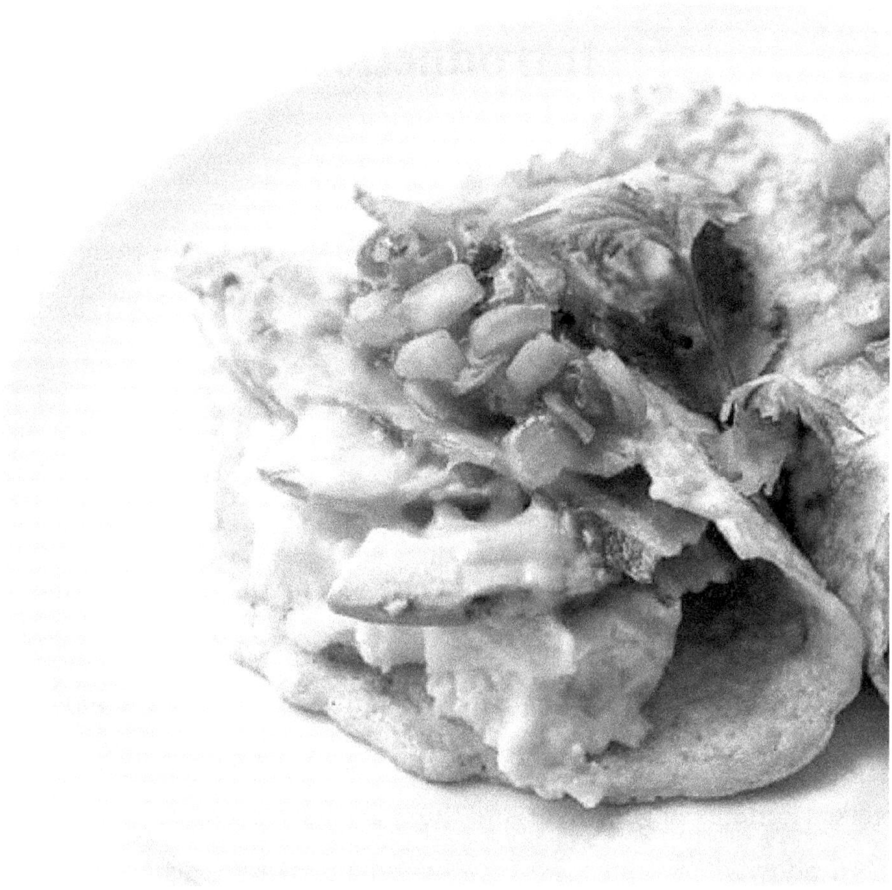

Introduction

Do you want to make a change in your life? Do you want to become a healthier person who can enjoy a new and improved life? Then, you are definitely in the right place. You are about to discover a wonderful and very healthy diet that has changed millions of lives. We are talking about the Ketogenic diet, a lifestyle that will mesmerize you and that will make you a new person in no time. So, let's sit back, relax and find out more about the Ketogenic diet.

A keto diet is a low carb one. This is the first and one of the most important things you should now. During such a diet, your body makes ketones in your liver and these are used as energy.
Your body will produce less insulin and glucose and a state of ketosis is induced.
Ketosis is a natural process that appears when our food intake is lower than usual. The body will soon adapt to this state and therefore you will be able to lose weight in no time but you will also become healthier and your physical and mental performances will improve.
Your blood sugar levels will improve and you won't be predisposed to diabetes.

Also, epilepsy and heart diseases can be prevented if you are on a Ketogenic diet.
Your cholesterol will improve and you will feel amazing in no time.
How does that sound?

A Ketogenic diet is simple and easy to follow as long as you follow some simple rules. You don't need to make huge changes but there are some things you should know.
So, here goes!

The list of foods you are allowed to eat during a keto diet is permissive and rich as you can see for yourself.
So, we think it should be pretty easy for you to start such a diet.

If you've made this choice already, then, it's time you checked our amazing keto recipe collection.
In this guide you will discover 50 of the best Breakfast and Lunch Ketogenic recipes in the world and you will soon be able to make each and every one of these recipes.

Now let's start our magical culinary journey!
Ketogenic lifestyle...here we come!
Enjoy!

Ketogenic Recipes For Breakfast

Amazing Breakfast In A Glass

Don't bother making something complex for breakfast! Try this amazing keto drink!

Preparation time: 3 minutes

Cooking time: 0 minutes

Servings: 2

Ingredients:

- 10 ounces canned coconut milk
- 1 cup favorite greens
- ¼ cup cocoa nibs
- 1 cup water
- 1 cup cherries, frozen
- ¼ cup cocoa powder
- 1 small avocado, pitted and peeled
- ¼ teaspoon turmeric

Directions:

1. In your blender, mix coconut milk with avocado, cocoa powder, cherries and turmeric and blend well.
2. Add water, greens and cocoa nibs, blend for 2 minutes more, pour into glasses and serve.

Enjoy!

Nutrition: calories 100, fat 3, fiber 2, carbs 3, protein 5

Delicious Chicken Quiche

It's so delicious that you will ask for more!

Preparation time: 10 minutes

Cooking time: 45 minutes

Servings: 5

Ingredients:

- 7 eggs
- 2 cups almond flour
- 2 tablespoons coconut oil
- Salt and black pepper to the taste
- 2 zucchinis, grated
- ½ cup heavy cream
- 1 teaspoon fennel seeds
- 1 teaspoon oregano, dried
- 1 pound chicken meat, ground

Directions:

1. In your food processor, blend almond flour with a pinch of salt.
2. Add 1 egg and coconut oil and blend well.

3. Place dough in a greased pie pan and press well on the bottom.
4. Heat up a pan over medium heat, add chicken meat, brown for a couple of minutes, take off heat and leave aside.
5. In a bowl, mix 6 eggs with salt, pepper, oregano, cream and fennel seeds and whisk well.
6. Add chicken meat and stir again.
7. Pour this into pie crust, spread, introduce in the oven at 350 degrees F and bake for 40 minutes.
8. Leave the pie to cool down a bit before slicing and serving it for breakfast!

Enjoy!

Nutrition: calories 300, fat 23, fiber 3, carbs 4, protein 18

Delicious Steak And Eggs

This is so rich and hearty! Dare and try this for breakfast tomorrow!

Preparation time: 10 minutes

Cooking time: 10 minutes

Servings: 1

Ingredients:

- 4 ounces sirloin
- 1 small avocado, pitted, peeled and sliced
- 3 eggs
- 1 tablespoon ghee
- Salt and black pepper to the taste

Directions:

1. Heat up a pan with the ghee over medium high heat, crack eggs into the pan and cook them as you wish.
2. Season with salt and pepper, take off heat and transfer to a plate.
3. Heat up another pan over medium high heat, add sirloin, cook for 4 minutes, take off heat, leave aside to cool down and cut into thin strips.

4. Season with salt and pepper to the taste and place next to the eggs.
5. Add avocado slices on the side and serve.

Enjoy!

Nutrition: calories 500, fat 34, fiber 10, carbs 3, protein 40

Amazing Chicken Omelet

It tastes amazing and it looks incredible! It's perfect!

Preparation time: 10 minutes

Cooking time: 10 minutes

Servings: 1

Ingredients:

- 1 ounce rotisserie chicken, shredded
- 1 teaspoon mustard
- 1 tablespoon homemade mayonnaise
- 1 tomato, chopped
- 2 bacon slices, cooked and crumbled
- 2 eggs
- 1 small avocado, pitted, peeled and chopped
- Salt and black pepper to the taste

Directions:

1. In a bowl, mix eggs with some salt and pepper and whisk gently.
2. Heat up a pan over medium heat, spray with some cooking oil, add eggs and cook your omelet for 5 minutes.

3. Add chicken, avocado, tomato, bacon, mayo and mustard on one half of the omelet.
4. Fold omelet, cover pan and cook for 5 minutes more.
5. Transfer to a plate and serve.

Enjoy!

Nutrition: calories 400, fat 32, fiber 6, carbs 4, protein 25

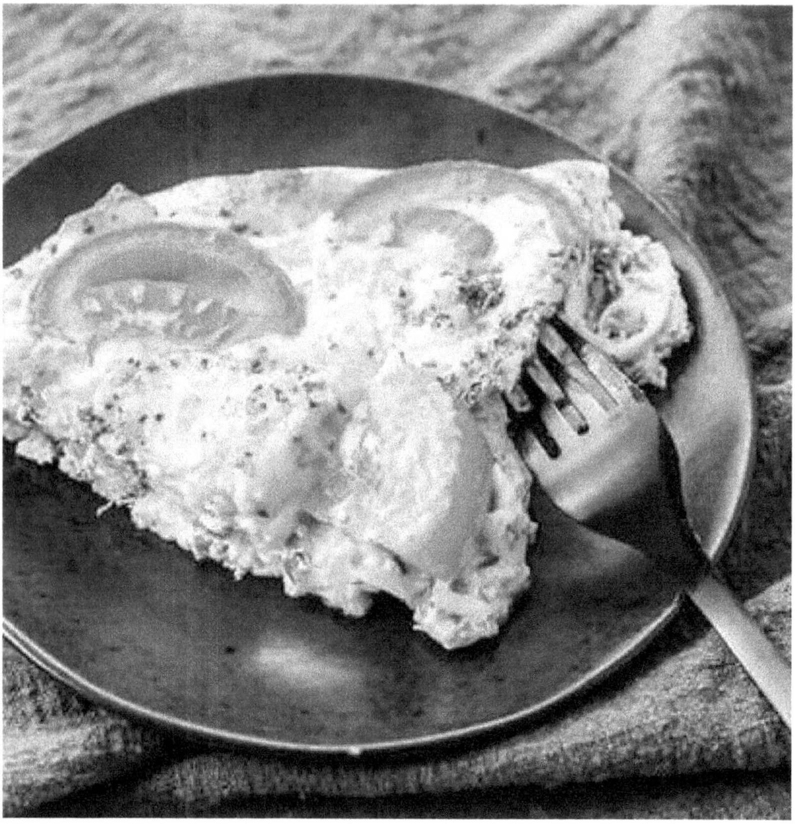

Simple Smoothie Bowl

It's one of the best keto breakfast ideas ever!

Preparation time: 5 minutes

Cooking time: 0 minutes

Servings: 1

Ingredients:

- 2 ice cubes
- 1 tablespoon coconut oil
- 2 tablespoons heavy cream
- 1 cup spinach
- ½ cup almond milk
- 1 teaspoon protein powder
- 4 raspberries
- 1 tablespoon coconut ,shredded
- 4 walnuts
- 1 teaspoon chia seeds

Directions:

1. In your blender, mix milk with spinach, cream, ice, protein powder and coconut oil, blend well and transfer to a bowl.

2. Top your bowl with raspberries, coconut, walnuts and chia seeds and serve.

Enjoy!

Nutrition: calories 450, fat 34, fiber 4, carbs 4, protein 35

Feta Omelet

The combination of ingredients is just wonderful!

Preparation time: 10 minutes

Cooking time: 10 minutes

Servings: 1

Ingredients:

- 3 eggs
- 1 tablespoon ghee
- 1 ounce feta cheese, crumbled
- 1 tablespoon heavy cream
- 1 tablespoon jarred pesto
- Salt and black pepper to the taste

Directions:

1. In a bowl, mix eggs with heavy cream, salt and pepper and whisk well.
2. Heat up a pan with the ghee over medium high heat, add whisked eggs, spread into the pan and cook your omelet until it's fluffy.
3. Sprinkle cheese and spread pesto on your omelet, fold in half, cover pan and cook for 5 minutes more.

4. Transfer omelet to a plate and serve.

Enjoy!

Nutrition: calories 500, fat 43, fiber 6, carbs 3, protein 30

Breakfast Meatloaf

This is something worth trying as soon as possible!

Preparation time: 10 minutes

Cooking time: 35 minutes

Servings: 4

Ingredients:

- 1 teaspoon ghee
- 1 small yellow onion, chopped
- 1 pound sweet sausage, chopped
- 6 eggs
- 1 cup cheddar cheese, shredded
- 4 ounces cream cheese, soft
- Salt and black pepper to the taste
- 2 tablespoons scallions, chopped

Directions:

1. In a bowl, mix eggs with salt, pepper, onion, sausage and half of the cream and whisk well.
2. Grease a meatloaf with the ghee, pour sausage and eggs mix, introduce in the oven at 350 degrees F and bake for 30 minutes.

3. Take meatloaf out of the oven, leave aside for a couple of minutes, spread the rest of the cream cheese on top and sprinkle scallions and cheddar cheese all over.
4. Introduce meatloaf in the oven again and bake for 5 minutes more.
5. After the time has passed, broil meatloaf for 3 minutes, leave it aside to cool down a bit, slice and serve it.

Enjoy!

Nutrition: calories 560, fat 32, fiber 1, carbs 6, protein 45

Breakfast Tuna Salad

You will love this Ketogenic breakfast from now on!

Preparation time: 10 minutes

Cooking time: 0 minutes

Servings: 4

Ingredients:

- 2 tablespoons sour cream
- 12 ounces tuna in olive oil
- 4 leeks, finely chopped
- Salt and black pepper to the taste
- A pinch of chili flakes
- 1 tablespoon capers
- 8 tablespoons homemade mayonnaise

Directions:

1. In a salad bowl, mix tuna with capers, salt, pepper, leeks, chili flakes, sour cream and mayo.
2. Stir well and serve with some crispy bread.

Enjoy!

Nutrition: calories 160, fat 2, fiber 1, carbs 2, protein 6

Incredible Breakfast Salad In A Jar

You can even take this at the office!

Preparation time: 10 minutes

Cooking time: 0 minutes

Servings: 1

Ingredients:

- 1 ounce favorite greens
- 1 ounce red bell pepper, chopped
- 1 ounce cherry tomatoes, halved
- 4 ounces rotisserie chicken, roughly chopped
- 4 tablespoons extra virgin olive oil
- ½ scallion, chopped
- 1 ounce cucumber, chopped
- Salt and black pepper to the taste

Directions:

1. In a bowl, mix greens with bell pepper, tomatoes, scallion, cucumber, salt, pepper and olive oil and toss to coat well.
2. Transfer this to a jar, top with chicken pieces and serve for breakfast.

Enjoy!

Nutrition: calories 180, fat 12, fiber 4, carbs 5, protein 17

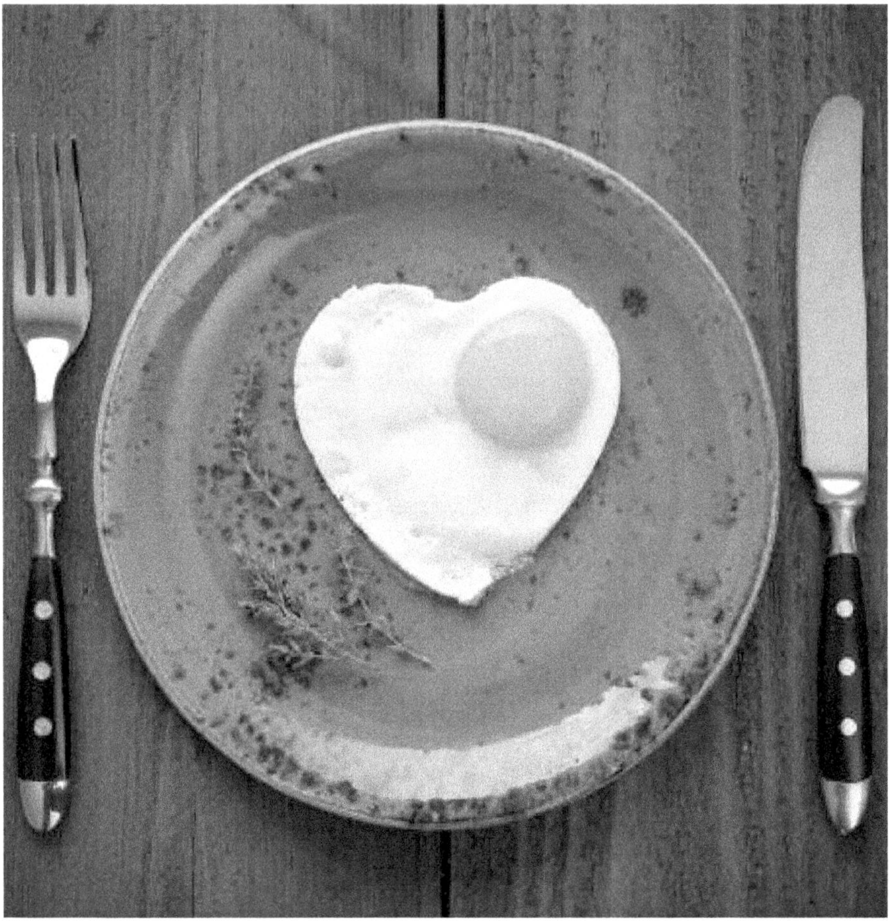

Delicious Naan Bread And Butter

Try this special keto breakfast! It's so easy to make!

Preparation time: 10 minutes

Cooking time: 10 minutes

Servings: 6

Ingredients:

- 7 tablespoons coconut oil
- ¾ cup coconut flour
- 2 tablespoons psyllium powder
- ½ teaspoon baking powder
- Salt to the taste
- 2 cups hot water
- Some coconut oil for frying
- 2 garlic cloves, minced
- 3.5 ounces ghee

Directions:

1. In a bowl, mix coconut flour with baking powder, salt and psyllium powder and stir.
2. Add 7 tablespoons coconut oil and the hot water and start kneading your dough.

3. Leave aside for 5 minutes, divide into 6 balls and flatten them on a working surface.
4. Heat up a pan with some coconut oil over medium high heat, add naan breads to the pan, fry them until they are golden and transfer them to a plate.
5. Heat up a pan with the ghee over medium high heat, add garlic, salt and pepper, stir and cook for 2 minutes.
6. Brush naan breads with this mix and pour the rest into a bowl.
7. Serve in the morning.

Enjoy!

Nutrition: calories 140, fat 9, fiber 2, carbs 3, protein 4

Ketogenic Recipes For Lunch

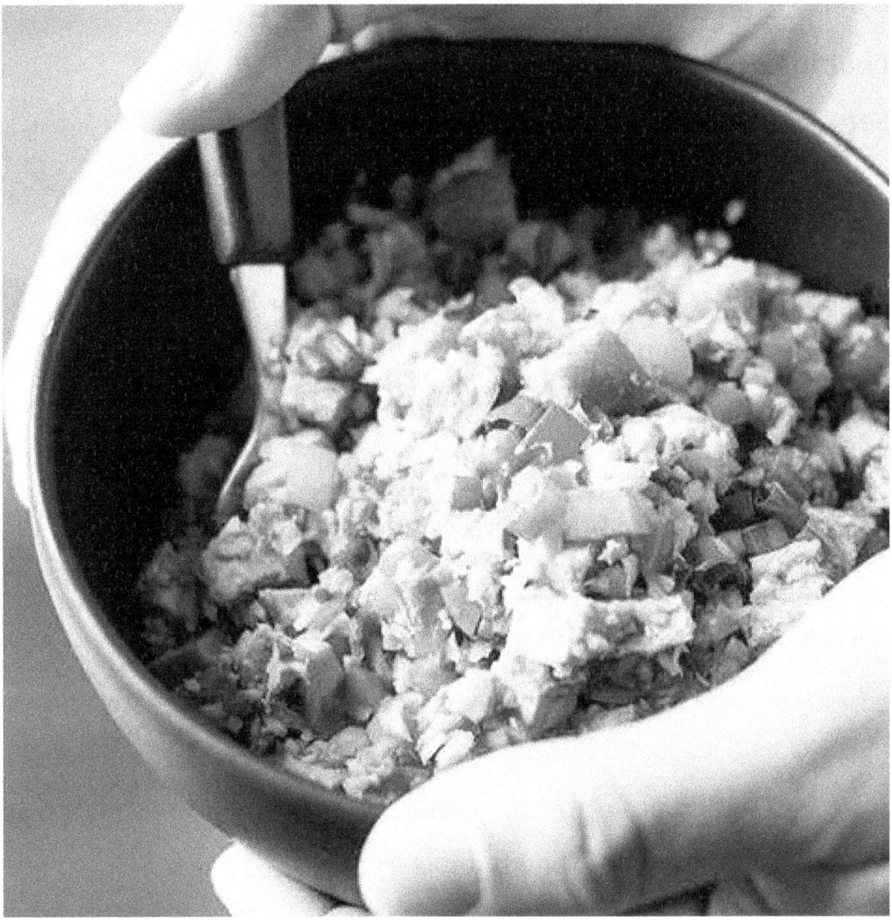

Lunch Caesar Salad

This is packed with healthy elements and it's 100% keto!

Preparation time: 10 minutes

Cooking time: 0 minutes

Servings: 2

Ingredients:

- 1 avocado, pitted, peeled and sliced
- Salt and black pepper to the taste
- 3 tablespoons creamy Caesar dressing
- 1 cup bacon, cooked and crumbled
- 1 chicken breast, grilled and shredded

Directions:

1. In a salad bowl, mix avocado with bacon and chicken breast and stir.
2. Add Caesar dressing, salt and pepper, toss to coat, divide into 2 bowls and serve.

Enjoy!

Nutrition: calories 334, fat 23, fiber 4, carbs 3, protein 18

Lunch Tacos

It's an easy and tasty lunch idea for all those who are on a Keto diet!

Preparation time: 10 minutes

Cooking time: 25 minutes

Servings: 3

Ingredients:

- 2 cups cheddar cheese, grated
- 1 small avocado, pitted, peeled and chopped
- 1 cup favorite taco meat, cooked
- 2 teaspoons sriracha sauce
- ¼ cup tomatoes, chopped
- Cooking spray
- Salt and black pepper to the taste

Directions:

1. Spray some cooking oil on lined baking dish.
2. Spread cheddar cheese on the baking sheet, introduce in the oven at 400 degrees F and bake for 15 minutes.
3. Spread taco meat over cheese and bake for 10 minutes more.

4. Meanwhile, in a bowl, mix avocado with tomatoes, sriracha sauce, salt and pepper and stir.
5. Spread this over taco and cheddar layers, leave tacos to cool down a bit, slice using a pizza slicer and serve for lunch.

Enjoy!

Nutrition: calories 400, fat 23, fiber 0, carbs 2, protein 37

Delicious Lunch Pizza

We recommend you to try this Ketogenic pizza for lunch today!

Preparation time: 10 minutes

Cooking time: 7 minutes

Servings: 4

Ingredients:

- 1 cup pizza cheese mix, shredded
- 1 tablespoon olive oil
- 2 tablespoons ghee
- 1 cup mozzarella cheese, shredded
- ¼ cup mascarpone cheese
- 1 tablespoon heavy cream
- 1 teaspoon garlic, minced
- Salt and black pepper to the taste
- A pinch of lemon pepper
- 1/3 cup broccoli florets, steamed
- Some asiago cheese, shaved for serving

Directions:

1. Heat up a pan with the oil over medium heat, add pizza cheese mix and spread into a circle.

2. Add mozzarella cheese and also spread into a circle.
3. Cook everything for 5 minutes and transfer to a plate.
4. Heat up the pan with the ghee over medium heat, add mascarpone cheese, cream, salt, pepper, lemon pepper and garlic, stir and cook for 5 minutes.
5. Drizzle half of this mix over cheese crust.
6. Add broccoli florets to the pan with the rest of the mascarpone mix, stir and cook for 1 minute.
7. Add this on top of the pizza, sprinkle asiago cheese at the end and serve.

Enjoy!

Nutrition: calories 250, fat 15, fiber 1, carbs 3, protein 10

Simple Pizza Rolls

These taste so divine! They are so amazing!

Preparation time: 10 minutes

Cooking time: 30 minutes

Servings: 6

Ingredients:

- ¼ cup mixed red and green bell peppers, chopped
- 2 cup mozzarella cheese, shredded
- 1 teaspoon pizza seasoning
- 2 tablespoons onion, chopped
- 1 tomato, chopped
- Salt and black pepper to the taste
- ¼ cup pizza sauce
- ½ cup sausage, crumbled and cooked

Directions:

1. Spread mozzarella cheese on a lined and lightly greased baking sheet, sprinkle pizza seasoning on top, introduce in the oven at 400 degrees F and bake for 20 minutes.

2. Take your pizza crust out of the oven, spread sausage, onion, bell peppers and tomatoes all over and drizzle the tomato sauce at the end.
3. Introduce in the oven again and bake for 10 minutes more.
4. Take pizza out of the oven, leave aside for a couple of minutes, slice into 6 pieces, roll each piece and serve for lunch!

Enjoy!

Nutrition: calories 117, fat 7, fiber 1, carbs 2, protein 11

Delicious Lunch Dish

Get all the ingredients you need and make this amazing keto lunch as soon as possible!

Preparation time: 10 minutes

Cooking time: 15 minutes

Servings: 2

Ingredients:

- 1 and ½ cups cheddar cheese, shredded
- 1 and ½ cups cheese blend
- 2 beef hot dogs, finely chopped
- A drizzle of olive oil
- 1 pound beef meat, ground
- Salt and black pepper to the taste
- ¼ teaspoon paprika
- ¼ teaspoon old bay
- ¼ teaspoon onion powder
- ¼ teaspoon garlic powder
- 1 cup lettuce leaves, chopped
- 1 tablespoon thousand island dressing
- 2 tablespoons dill pickle, chopped
- 2 tablespoons yellow onion, chopped
- ½ cup American cheese, shredded

- Some ketchup for serving
- Some mustard for serving

Directions:

1. Heat up a pan with a drizzle of oil over medium heat, add half of the cheese blend, spread into a circle and top with half of the cheddar cheese.
2. Also spread into a circle, cook for 5 minutes, transfer to a cutting board and leave aside for a few minutes to cool down.
3. Heat up the pan again, add the rest of the cheese blend and spread into a circle.
4. Add the rest of the cheddar, also spread, cook for 5 minutes and also transfer to a cutting board.
5. Spread the thousand island dressing over the 2 pizza crusts.
6. Heat up the same pan again over medium heat, add beef, stir and brown for a few minutes.
7. Add salt, pepper, old bay seasoning, paprika, onion and garlic powder, stir and cook for a few minutes more.
8. Add hot dogs pieces, stir and cook for 5 minutes more.
9. Spread lettuce, pickles, American cheese and onions on the 2 pizza crusts.
10. Divide beef and hot dog mix, drizzle mustard and ketchup at the end and serve.

Nutrition: calories 200, fat 6, fiber 3, carbs 1.5, protein 10

Delicious Mexican Lunch

It's so delicious! Why don't you try it today?

Preparation time: 10 minutes

Cooking time: 20 minutes

Servings: 4

Ingredients:

- ¼ cup cilantro, chopped
- 2 avocados, pitted, peeled and cut into chunks
- 1 tablespoon lime juice
- ¼ cup white onion, chopped
- 1 teaspoon garlic, minced
- Salt and black pepper to the taste
- 6 cherry tomatoes, cut in quarters
- ½ cup water
- 2-pound beef meat, ground
- 2 cups sour cream
- ¼ cup taco seasoning
- 2 cups lettuce leaves, shredded
- Some cayenne pepper sauce for serving
- 2 cups cheddar cheese, shredded

Directions:

1. In a bowl, mix cilantro with lime juice, avocado, onion, tomatoes, salt, pepper and garlic, stir well and leave aside in the fridge for now.
2. Heat up a pan over medium heat, add beef, stir and brown for 10 minutes.
3. Add taco seasoning and water, stir and cook over medium-low heat for 10 minutes more.
4. Divide this mix into 4 serving bowls.
5. Add sour cream, avocado mix you've made earlier, lettuce pieces and cheddar cheese.
6. Drizzle cayenne pepper sauce at the end and serve for lunch!

Enjoy!

Nutrition: calories 340, fat 30, fiber 5, carbs 3, protein 32

Lunch Stuffed Peppers

These are perfect for a Ketogenic lunch!

Preparation time: 10 minutes

Cooking time: 40 minutes

Servings: 4

Ingredients:

- 4 big banana peppers, tops cut off, seeds removed and cut into halves lengthwise
- 1 tablespoon ghee
- Salt and black pepper to the taste
- ½ teaspoon herbs de Provence
- 1 pound sweet sausage, chopped
- 3 tablespoons yellow onions, chopped
- Some marinara sauce
- A drizzle of olive oil

Directions:

1. Season banana peppers with salt and pepper, drizzle the oil, rub well and bake in the oven at 350 degrees F for 20 minutes.

2. Meanwhile, heat up a pan over medium heat, add sausage pieces, stir and cook for 5 minutes.
3. Add onion, herbs de Provence, salt, pepper and ghee, stir well and cook for 5 minutes.
4. Take peppers out of the oven, fill them with the sausage mix, place them in an oven-proof dish, drizzle marinara sauce over them, introduce in the oven again and bake for 10 minutes more.
5. Serve hot.

Enjoy!

Nutrition: calories 320, fat 8, fiber 4, carbs 3, protein 10

Special Lunch Burgers

These burgers are really something very special!

Preparation time: 10 minutes

Cooking time: 25 minutes

Servings: 8

Ingredients:

- 1 pound brisket, ground
- 1 pound beef, ground
- Salt and black pepper to the taste
- 8 butter slices
- 1 tablespoon garlic, minced
- 1 tablespoon Italian seasoning
- 2 tablespoons mayonnaise
- 1 tablespoon ghee
- 2 tablespoons olive oil
- 1 yellow onion, chopped
- 1 tablespoon water

Directions:

1. In a bowl, mix brisket with beef, salt, pepper, Italian seasoning, garlic and mayo and stir well.

2. Shape 8 patties and make a pocket in each.
3. Stuff each burger with a butter slice and seal.
4. Heat up a pan with the olive oil over medium heat, add onions, stir and cook for 2 minutes.
5. Add the water, stir and gather them in the corner of the pan.
6. Place burgers in the pan with the onions and cook them over medium-low heat for 10 minutes.
7. Flip them, add the ghee and cook them for 10 minutes more.
8. Divide burgers on buns and serve them with caramelized onions on top.

Enjoy!

Nutrition: calories 180, fat 8, fiber 1, carbs 4, protein 20

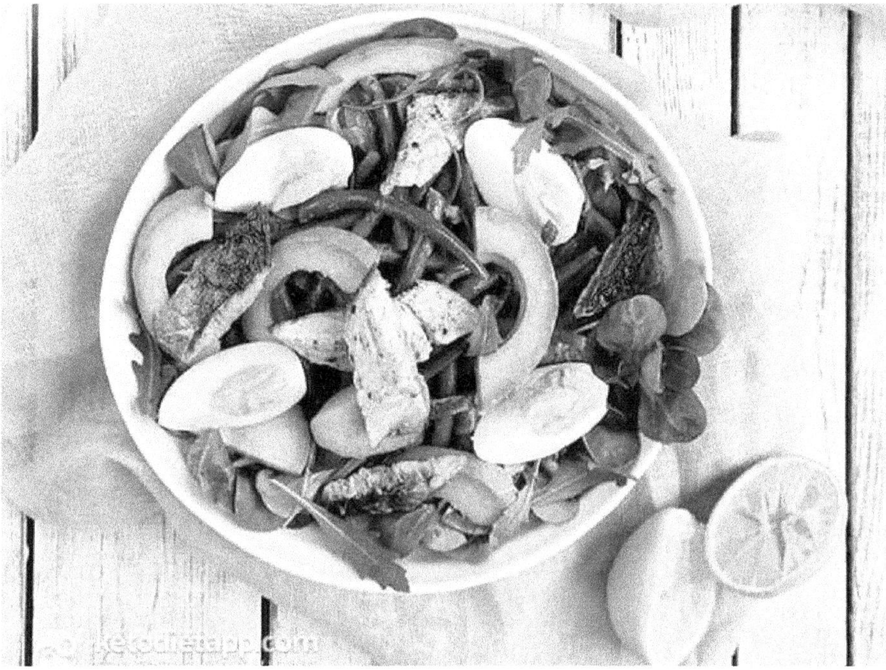
ketodietapp.com

Different Burger

serve this burger with the sauce we recommend you and enjoy!

Preparation time: 10 minutes

Cooking time: 30 minutes

Servings: 4

Ingredients:

For the sauce:

- 4 chili peppers, chopped
- 1 cup water
- 1 cup almond butter
- 1 teaspoon swerve
- 6 tablespoons coconut aminos
- 4 garlic cloves, minced
- 1 tablespoon rice vinegar

For the burgers:

- 4 pepper jack cheese slices
- 1 and ½ pounds beef, ground
- 1 red onion, sliced
- 8 bacon slices
- 8 lettuce leaves

- Salt and black pepper to the taste

Directions:

1. Heat up a pan with the almond butter over medium heat.
2. Add water, stir well and bring to a simmer.
3. Add coconut aminos and stir well.
4. In your food processor, mix chili peppers with garlic, swerve and vinegar and blend well.
5. Add this to almond butter mix, stir well, take off heat and leave aside for now.
6. In a bowl, mix beef with salt and pepper, stir and shape 4 patties.
7. Place them in a pan, introduce in your preheated broiler and broil for 7 minutes.
8. Flip burgers and broil them for 7 minutes more.
9. Place cheese slices on burgers, introduce in your broiler and broil for 4 minutes more.
10. Heat up a pan over medium heat, add bacon slices and fry them for a couple of minutes.
11. Place 2 lettuce leaves on a dish, add 1 burger on top, then 1 onion slice and 1 bacon slice and top with some almond butter sauce.
12. Repeat with the rest of the lettuce leaves, burgers, onion, bacon and sauce.

Enjoy!

Nutrition: calories 700, fat 56, fiber 10, carbs 7, protein 40

Delicious Zucchini Dish

It's easy to make and very light! Try this lunch dish soon!

Preparation time: 10 minutes

Cooking time: 5 minutes

Servings: 1

Ingredients:

- 1 tablespoon olive oil
- 3 tablespoons ghee
- 2 cups zucchini, cut with a spiralizer
- 1 teaspoon red pepper flakes
- 1 tablespoon garlic, minced
- 1 tablespoon red bell pepper, chopped
- Salt and black pepper to the taste
- 1 tablespoon basil, chopped
- ¼ cup asiago cheese, shaved
- ¼ cup parmesan, grated

Directions:

1. Heat up a pan with the oil and ghee over medium heat, add garlic, bell pepper and pepper flakes, stir and cook for 1 minute.

2. Add zucchini noodles, stir and cook for 2 minutes more.
3. Add basil, parmesan, salt and pepper, stir and cook for a few seconds more.
4. Take off heat, transfer to a bowl and serve for lunch with asiago cheese on top.

Enjoy!

Nutrition: calories 140, fat 3, fiber 1, carbs 1.3, protein 5

Bacon And Zucchini Noodles Salad

It's so refreshing and healthy! We adore this salad!

Preparation time: 10 minutes

Cooking time: 0 minutes

Servings: 2

Ingredients:

- 1 cup baby spinach
- 4 cups zucchini noodles
- 1/3 cup bleu cheese, crumbled
- 1/3 cup thick cheese dressing
- ½ cup bacon, cooked and crumbled
- Black pepper to the taste

Directions:

1. In a salad bowl, mix spinach with zucchini noodles, bacon and bleu cheese and toss.
2. Add cheese dressing and black pepper to the taste, toss well to coat, divide into 2 bowls and serve.

Enjoy!

Nutrition: calories 200, fat 14, fiber 4, carbs 2, protein 10

Amazing Chicken Salad

The best chicken salad you could taste is now available for you!

Preparation time: 10 minutes

Cooking time: 0 minutes

Servings: 3

Ingredients:

- 1 green onion, chopped
- 1 celery rib, chopped
- 1 egg, hard-boiled, peeled and chopped
- 5 ounces chicken breast, roasted and chopped
- 2 tablespoons parsley, chopped
- ½ tablespoons dill relish
- Salt and black pepper to the taste
- 1/3 cup mayonnaise
- A pinch of granulated garlic
- 1 teaspoon mustard

Directions:

1. In your food processor, mix parsley with onion and celery and pulse well.
2. Transfer these to a bowl and leave aside for now.

3. Put chicken meat in your food processor, blend well and add to the bowl with the veggies.
4. Add egg pieces, salt and pepper and stir.
5. Also add mustard, mayo, dill relish and granulated garlic, toss to coat and serve right away.

Enjoy!

Nutrition: calories 283, fat 23, fiber 5, carbs 3, protein 12

Unbelievable Steak Salad

If you are not in the mood for a Ketogenic chicken salad, then try a steak one instead!

Preparation time: 10 minutes

Cooking time: 20 minutes

Servings: 4

Ingredients:

- 1 and ½ pound steak, thinly sliced
- 3 tablespoons avocado oil
- Salt and black pepper to the taste
- ¼ cup balsamic vinegar
- 6 ounces sweet onion, chopped
- 1 lettuce head, chopped
- 2 garlic cloves, minced
- 4 ounces mushrooms, sliced
- 1 avocado, pitted, peeled and sliced
- 3 ounces sun-dried tomatoes, chopped
- 1 yellow bell pepper, sliced
- 1 orange bell pepper, sliced
- 1 teaspoon Italian seasoning

- 1 teaspoon red pepper flakes
- 1 teaspoon onion powder

Directions:

1. In a bowl, mix steak pieces with some salt, pepper and balsamic vinegar, toss to coat and leave aside for now.
2. Heat up a pan with the avocado oil over medium-low heat, add mushrooms, garlic, salt, pepper and onion, stir and cook for 20 minutes.
3. In a bowl, mix lettuce leaves with orange and yellow bell pepper, sun dried tomatoes and avocado and stirred.
4. Season steak pieces with onion powder, pepper flakes and Italian seasoning.
5. Place steak pieces in a broiling pan, introduce in preheated broiler and cook for 5 minutes.
6. Divide steak pieces on plates, add lettuce and avocado salad on the side and top everything with onion and mushroom mix.

Enjoy!

Nutrition: calories 435, fat 23, fiber 7, carbs 10, protein 35

Fennel and Chicken Lunch Salad

Try each day a different lunch salad! Today, we suggest you try this fennel and chicken delight!

Preparation time: 10 minutes

Cooking time: 0 minutes

Servings: 4

Ingredients:

- 3 chicken breasts, boneless, skinless, cooked and chopped
- 2 tablespoons walnut oil
- ¼ cup walnuts, toasted and chopped
- 1 and ½ cup fennel, chopped
- 2 tablespoons lemon juice
- ¼ cup mayonnaise
- 2 tablespoons fennel fronds, chopped
- Salt and black pepper to the taste
- A pinch of cayenne pepper

Directions:

1. In a bowl, mix fennel with chicken and walnuts and stir.
2. In another bowl, mix mayo with salt, pepper, fennel fronds, walnut oil, lemon juice, cayenne and garlic and stir well.
3. Pour this over chicken and fennel mix, toss to coat well and keep in the fridge until you serve.

Enjoy!

Nutrition: calories 200, fat 10, fiber 1, carbs 3, protein 7

Easy Stuffed Avocado

it's so easy to make for lunch!

Preparation time: 10 minutes

Cooking time: 0 minutes

Servings: 1

Ingredients:

- 1 avocado
- 4 ounces canned sardines, drained
- 1 spring onion, chopped
- 1 tablespoon mayonnaise
- 1 tablespoon lemon juice
- Salt and black pepper to the taste
- ¼ teaspoon turmeric powder

Directions:

1. Cut avocado in halves, scoop flesh and put in a bowl.
2. Mash with a fork and mix with sardines.
3. Mash again with your fork and mix with onion, lemon juice, turmeric powder, salt, pepper and mayo.

4. Stir everything and divide into avocado halves.
5. Serve for lunch right away.

Enjoy!

Nutrition: calories 230, fat 34, fiber 12, carbs 5, protein 27

Pesto Chicken Salad

The combination is absolutely delicious! You should try it!

Preparation time: 10 minutes

Cooking time: 0 minutes

Servings: 4

Ingredients:

- 1 pound chicken meat, cooked and cubed
- Salt and black pepper to the taste
- 10 cherry tomatoes, halved
- 6 bacon slices, cooked and crumbled
- ¼ cup mayonnaise
- 1 avocado, pitted, peeled and cubed
- 2 tablespoons garlic pesto

Directions:

1. In a salad bowl, mix chicken with bacon, avocado, tomatoes, salt and pepper and stir.
2. Add mayo and garlic pesto, toss well to coat and serve.

Enjoy!

Nutrition: calories 357, fat 23, fiber 5, carbs 3, protein 26

Tasty Lunch Salad

It's delicious and you will adore it once you try it!

Preparation time: 10 minutes

Cooking time: 10 minutes

Servings: 1

Ingredients:

- 4 ounces beef steak
- 2 cups lettuce leaves, shredded
- Salt and black pepper to the taste
- Cooking spray
- 2 tablespoons cilantro, chopped
- 2 radishes, sliced
- 1/3 cup red cabbage, shredded
- 3 tablespoons jarred chimichurri sauce
- 1 tablespoons salad dressing

For the salad dressing:

- 3 garlic cloves, minced
- ½ teaspoon Worcestershire sauce
- 1 tablespoon mustard
- ½ cup apple cider vinegar

- ¼ cup water
- ½ cup olive oil
- ¼ teaspoon Tabasco sauce
- Salt and black pepper to the taste

Directions:

1. In a bowl, mix garlic cloves with Worcestershire sauce, mustard, cider vinegar, water, olive oil, salt, pepper and Tabasco sauce, whisk well and leave aside for now.
2. Heat up your kitchen grill over medium high heat, spray cooking oil, add steak, season with salt and pepper, cook for 4 minutes, flip, cook for 4 minutes more, take off heat, leave aside to cool down and cut into thin strips.
3. In a salad bowl, mix lettuce with cilantro, cabbage, radishes, chimichurri sauce and steak strips.
4. Add 1 tablespoons of salad dressing, toss to coat and serve right away.

Enjoy!

Nutrition: calories 456, fat 32, fiber 2, carbs 6, protein 30

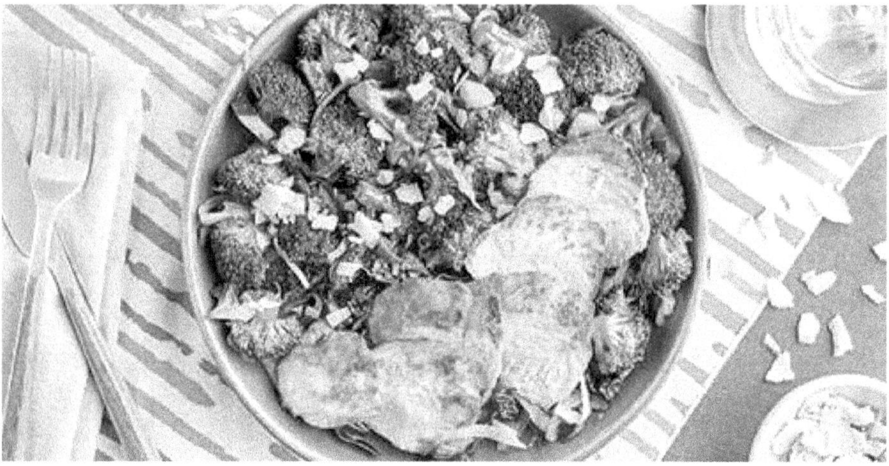

Easy Lunch Crab Cakes

Try these crab cakes for lunch! You won't regret it!

Preparation time: 10 minutes

Cooking time: 12 minutes

Servings: 6

Ingredients:

- 1 pound crabmeat
- ¼ cup parsley, chopped
- Salt and black pepper to the taste
- 2 green onions, chopped
- ¼ cup cilantro, chopped
- 1 teaspoon jalapeno pepper, minced
- 1 teaspoon lemon juice
- 1 teaspoon Worcestershire sauce
- 1 teaspoon old bay seasoning
- ½ teaspoon mustard powder
- ½ cup mayonnaise
- 1 egg
- 2 tablespoons olive oil

Directions:

1. In a large bowl mix crab meat with salt, pepper, parsley, green onions, cilantro, jalapeno, lemon juice, old bay seasoning, mustard powder and Worcestershire sauce and stir very well.
2. In another bowl mix egg wit mayo and whisk.
3. Add this to crabmeat mix and stir everything.
4. Shape 6 patties from this mix and place them on a plate.
5. Heat up a pan with the oil over medium high heat, add 3 crab cakes, cook for 3 minutes, flip, cook them for 3 minutes more and transfer to paper towels.
6. Repeat with the other 3 crab cakes, drain excess grease and serve for lunch.

Enjoy!

Nutrition: calories 254, fat 17, fiber 1, carbs 1, protein 20

Easy Lunch Muffins

These muffins will really get to your soul!

Preparation time: 10 minutes

Cooking time: 45 minutes

Servings: 13

Ingredients:

- 6 egg yolks
- 2 tablespoons coconut aminos
- ½ pound mushrooms
- ¾ cup coconut flour
- 1 pound beef, ground
- Salt to the taste

Directions:

1. In your food processor, mix mushrooms with salt, coconut aminos and egg yolks and blend well.
2. In a bowl, mix beef meat with some salt and stir.
3. Add mushroom mix to beef and stir everything.
4. Add coconut flour and stir again.
5. Divide this into 13 cupcake cups, introduce in the oven at 350 degrees f and bake for 45 minutes.

6. Serve them for lunch!

Enjoy!

Nutrition: calories 160, fat 10, fiber 3, carbs 1, protein 12

Lunch Pork Pie

This is something you've been craving for a very long time! Don't worry! It's a keto idea!

Preparation time: 10 minutes

Cooking time: 50 minutes

Servings: 6

Ingredients:

For the pie crust:

- 2 cups cracklings
- ¼ cup flax meal
- 1 cup almond flour
- 2 eggs
- A pinch of salt

For the filling:

- 1 cup cheddar cheese, grated
- 4 eggs
- 12 ounces pork loin, chopped
- 6 bacon slices
- ½ cup cream cheese
- 1 red onion, chopped

- ¼ cup chives, chopped
- 2 garlic cloves, minced
- Salt and black pepper to the taste
- 2 tablespoons ghee

Directions:

1. In your food processor, mix cracklings with almond flour, flax meal, 2 eggs and salt and blend until you obtain a dough.
2. Transfer this to a pie pan and press well on the bottom.
3. Introduce in the oven at 350 degrees F and bake for 15 minutes.
4. Meanwhile, heat up a pan with the ghee over medium high heat, add garlic and onion, stir and cook for 5 minutes.
5. Add bacon, stir and cook for 5 minutes.
6. Add pork loin, cook until it's brown on all sides and take off heat.
7. In a bowl, mix eggs with salt, pepper, cheddar cheese and cream cheese and blend well.
8. Add chives and stir again.
9. Spread pork into pie pan, add eggs mix, introduce in the oven at 350 degrees F and bake for 25 minutes.

10. Leave the pie to cool down for a couple of minutes and serve.

Enjoy!

Nutrition: calories 455, fat 34, fiber 3, carbs 3, protein 33

Delicious Lunch Pate

Enjoy something really easy to launch: a Ketogenic liver pate!

Preparation time: 10 minutes

Cooking time: 0 minutes

Servings: 1

Ingredients:

- 4 ounces chicken livers, sautéed
- 1 teaspoon mixed thyme, sage and oregano, chopped
- Salt and black pepper to the taste
- 3 tablespoons butter
- 3 radishes, thinly sliced
- Crusted bread slices for serving

Directions:

1. In your food processor, mix chicken livers with thyme, sage, oregano, butter, salt and pepper and blend very well for a few minutes.
2. Spread on crusted bread slices and top with radishes slices.
3. Serve right away.

Enjoy!

Nutrition: calories 380, fat 40, fiber 5, carbs 1, protein 17

Delicious Lunch Chowder

You might end up adoring this chowder! Try it at least once!

Preparation time: 10 minutes

Cooking time: 4 hours

Servings: 4

Ingredients:

- 1 pound chicken thighs, skinless and boneless
- 10 ounces canned tomatoes, chopped
- 1 cup chicken stock
- 8 ounces cream cheese
- Juice from 1 lime
- Salt and black pepper to the taste
- 1 jalapeno pepper, chopped
- 1 yellow onion, chopped
- 2 tablespoons cilantro, chopped
- 1 garlic clove, minced
- Cheddar cheese, shredded for serving
- Lime wedges for serving

Directions:

1. In your crock pot, mix chicken with tomatoes, stock, cream cheese, salt, pepper, lime juice, jalapeno, onion, garlic and cilantro, stir, cover and cook on High for 4 hours.
2. Uncover pot, shred meat into the pot, divide into bowls and serve with cheddar cheese on top and lime wedges on the side.

Enjoy!

Nutrition: calories 300, fat 5, fiber 6, carbs 3, protein 26

Delicious Coconut Soup

Try this Ketogenic coconut soup really soon! Everyone will love it!

Preparation time: 10 minutes

Cooking time: 30 minutes

Servings: 2

Ingredients:

- 4 cups chicken stock
- 3 lime leaves
- 1 and ½ cups coconut milk
- 1 teaspoon lemongrass, dried
- 1 cup cilantro, chopped
- 1 inch ginger, grated
- 4 Thai chilies, dried and chopped
- Salt and black pepper to the taste
- 4 ounces shrimp, raw, peeled and deveined
- 2 tablespoons red onion, chopped
- 1 tablespoon coconut oil
- 2 tablespoons mushrooms, chopped
- 1 tablespoon fish sauce
- 1 tablespoon cilantro, chopped

- Juice from 1 lime

Directions:

1. In a pot, mix chicken stock with coconut milk, lime leaves, lemongrass, Thai chilies, 1 cup cilantro, ginger, salt and pepper, stir, bring to a simmer over medium heat, cook for 20 minutes, strain and return to pot.
2. Heat up soup again over medium heat, add coconut oil, shrimp, fish sauce, mushrooms and onions, stir and cook for 10 minutes more.
3. Add lime juice and 1 tablespoon cilantro, stir, ladle into bowls and serve for lunch!

Enjoy!

Nutrition: calories 450, fat 34, fiber 4, carbs 8, protein 12

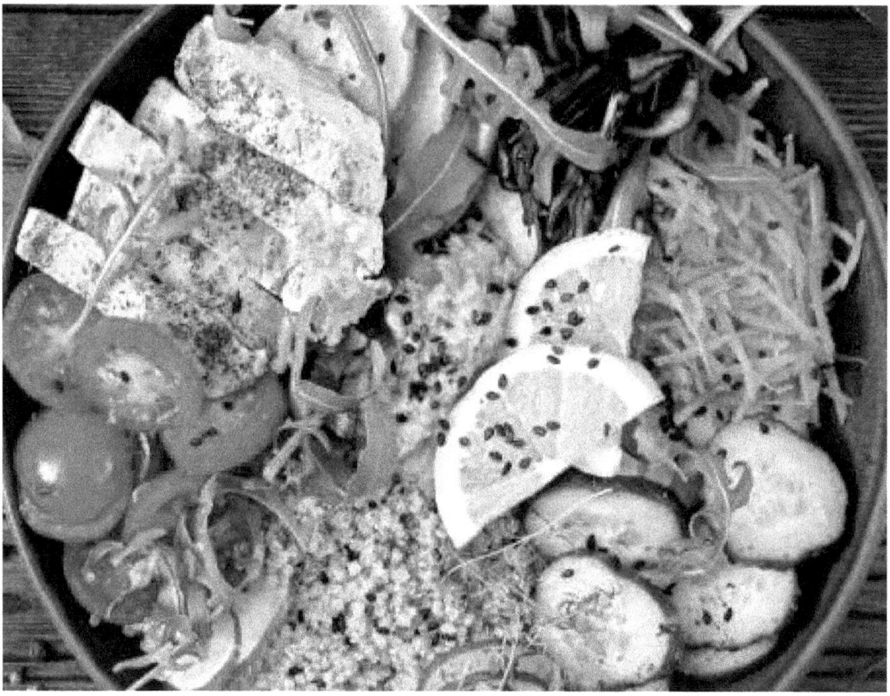

Zucchini Noodles Soup

This Ketogenic soup is simple and very tasty!

Preparation time: 10 minutes

Cooking time: 15 minutes

Servings: 8

Ingredients:

- 1 small yellow onion, chopped
- 2 garlic cloves, minced
- 1 jalapeno pepper, chopped
- 1 tablespoon coconut oil
- 1 and ½ tablespoons curry paste
- 6 cups chicken stock
- 15 ounces canned coconut milk
- 1 pound chicken breasts, sliced
- 1 red bell pepper, sliced
- 2 tablespoons fish sauce
- 2 zucchinis, cut with a spiralizer
- ½ cup cilantro, chopped
- Lime wedges for serving

Directions:

1. Heat up a pot with the oil over medium heat, add onion, stir and cook for 5 minutes.
2. Add garlic, jalapeno and curry paste, stir and cook for 1 minute.
3. Add stock and coconut milk, stir and bring to a boil.
4. Add red bell pepper, chicken and fish sauce, stir and simmer for 4 minutes more.
5. Add cilantro, stir, cook for 1 minute and take off heat.
6. Divide zucchini noodles into soup bowls, add soup on top and serve with lime wedges on the side.

Enjoy!

Nutrition: calories 287, fat 14, fiber 2, carbs 7, protein 25

Delicious Lunch Curry

Have you ever tried a keto curry? Then pay attention next!

Preparation time: 10 minutes

Cooking time: 1 hour

Servings: 4

Ingredients:

- 3 tomatoes, chopped
- 2 tablespoons olive oil
- 1 cup chicken stock
- 14 ounces canned coconut milk
- 1 tablespoon lime juice
- Salt and black pepper to the taste
- 2 pounds chicken thighs, boneless and skinless and cubed
- 2 garlic cloves, minced
- 1 cup white onion, chopped
- 3 red chilies, chopped
- 1 ounce peanuts, toasted
- 1 tablespoon water
- 1 tablespoon ginger, grated

- 2 teaspoons coriander, ground
- 1 teaspoon cinnamon, ground
- 1 teaspoon turmeric, ground
- 1 teaspoon cumin, ground
- ½ teaspoon black pepper
- 1 teaspoon fennel seeds, ground

Directions:

1. In your food processor, mix white onion with garlic, peanuts, red chilies, water, ginger, coriander, cinnamon, turmeric, cumin, fennel and black pepper, blend until you obtain a paste and leave aside for now.
2. Heat up a pan with the olive oil over medium high heat, add spice paste you've made, stir well and heat up for a few seconds.
3. Add chicken pieces, stir and cook for 2 minutes.
4. Add stock and tomatoes, stir, reduce heat to low and cook for 30 minutes.
5. Add coconut milk, stir and cook for 20 minutes more.
6. Add salt, pepper and lime juice, stir, divide into bowls and serve.

Enjoy!

Nutrition: calories 430, fat 22, fiber 4, carbs 7, protein 53

Lunch Spinach Rolls

These will be ready in no time!

Preparation time: 20 minutes

Cooking time: 15 minutes

Servings: 16

Ingredients:

- 6 tablespoons coconut flour
- ½ cup almond flour
- 2 and ½ cups mozzarella cheese, shredded
- 2 eggs
- A pinch of salt

For the filling:

- 4 ounces cream cheese
- 6 ounces spinach, torn
- A drizzle of avocado oil
- A pinch of salt
- ¼ cup parmesan, grated
- Mayonnaise for serving

Directions:

1. Heat up a pan with the oil over medium heat, add spinach and cook for 2 minutes.
2. Add parmesan, a pinch of salt and cream cheese, stir well, take off heat and leave aside for now.
3. Put mozzarella cheese in a heatproof bowl and microwave for 30 seconds.
4. Add eggs, salt, coconut and almond flour and stir everything.
5. Place dough on a lined cutting board, place a parchment paper on top and flatten dough with a rolling pin.
6. Divide dough into 16 rectangles, spread spinach mix on each and roll them into cigar shapes.
7. Place all rolls on a lined baking sheet, introduce in the oven at 350 degrees F and bake for 15 minutes.
8. Leave rolls to cool down for a few minutes before serving them with some mayo on top.

Enjoy!

Nutrition: calories 500, fat 65, fiber 4, carbs 14, protein 32

Delicious Steak Bowl

It's an easy and fulfilling keto lunch! Try it!

Preparation time: 15 minutes

Cooking time: 8 minutes

Servings: 4

Ingredients:

- 16 ounces skirt steak
- 4 ounces pepper jack cheese, shredded
- 1 cup sour cream
- Salt and black pepper to the taste
- 1 handful cilantro, chopped
- A splash of chipotle adobo sauce

For the guacamole:

- ¼ cup red onion, chopped
- 2 avocados, pitted and peeled
- Juice from 1 lime
- 1 tablespoon olive oil
- 6 cherry tomatoes, chopped
- 1 garlic clove, minced
- 1 tablespoon cilantro, chopped

- Salt and black pepper to the taste

Directions:

1. Put avocados in a bowl and mash with a fork.
2. Add tomatoes, red onion, garlic, salt and pepper and stir well.
3. Add olive oil, lime juice and 1 tablespoon cilantro, stir again very well and leave aside for now.
4. Heat up a pan over high heat, add steak, season with salt and pepper, cook for 4 minutes on each side, transfer to a cutting board, leave aside to cool down a bit and cut into thin strips.
5. Divide steak into 4 bowls, add cheese, sour cream and guacamole on top and serve with a splash of chipotle adobo sauce.

Enjoy!

Nutrition: calories 600, fat 50, fiber 6, carbs 5, protein 30

Meatballs And Pilaf

This is a Ketogenic lunch everyone can enjoy!

Preparation time: 10 minutes

Cooking time: 30 minutes

Servings: 4

Ingredients:

- 12 ounces cauliflower florets
- Salt and black pepper to the taste
- 1 egg
- 1 pound lamb, ground
- 1 teaspoon fennel seed
- 1 teaspoon paprika
- 1 teaspoon garlic powder
- 1 small yellow onion, chopped
- 2 garlic cloves, minced
- 2 tablespoons coconut oil
- 1 bunch mint, chopped
- 1 tablespoon lemon zest
- 4 ounces goat cheese, crumbled

Directions:

1. Put cauliflower florets in your food processor, add salt and pulse well.
2. Grease a pan with some of the coconut oil, heat up over medium heat, add cauliflower rice, cook for 8 minutes, season with salt and pepper to the taste, take off heat and keep warm.
3. In a bowl, mix lamb with salt, pepper, egg, paprika, garlic powder and fennel seed and stir very well.
4. Shape 12 meatballs and place them on a plate for now.
5. Heat up a pan with the coconut oil over medium heat, add onion, stir and cook for 6 minutes.
6. Add garlic, stir and cook for 1 minute.
7. Add meatballs, cook them well on all sides and take off heat.
8. Divide cauliflower rice between plates, add meatballs and onion mix on top, sprinkle mint, lemon zest and goat cheese at the end and serve.

Enjoy!

Nutrition: calories 470, fat 43, fiber 5, carbs 4, protein 26

Delicious Broccoli Soup

Try this superb soup as soon as possible!

Preparation time: 10 minutes

Cooking time: 30 minutes

Servings: 4

Ingredients:

- 1 white onion, chopped
- 1 tablespoon ghee
- 2 cups veggie stock
- Salt and black pepper to the taste
- 2 cups water
- 2 garlic cloves, minced
- 1 cup heavy cream
- 8 ounces cheddar cheese, grated
- 12 ounces broccoli florets
- ½ teaspoon paprika

Directions:

1. Heat up a pot with the ghee over medium heat, add onion and garlic, stir and cook for 5 minutes.

2. Add stock, cream, water, salt, pepper and paprika, stir and bring to a boil.
3. Add broccoli, stir and simmer soup for 25 minutes.
4. Transfer to your food processor and blend well.
5. Add cheese and blend again.
6. Divide into soup bowls and serve hot.

Enjoy!

Nutrition: calories 350, fat 34, fiber 7, carbs 7, protein 11

Lunch Green Beans Salad

It will soon become one of your favorite keto salads!

Preparation time: 10 minutes

Cooking time: 5 minutes

Servings: 8

Ingredients:

- 2 tablespoons white wine vinegar
- 1 and ½ tablespoons mustard
- Salt and black pepper to the taste
- 2 pounds green beans
- 1/3 cup extra virgin olive oil
- 1 and ½ cups fennel, thinly sliced
- 4 ounces goat cheese, crumbled
- ¾ cup walnuts, toasted and chopped

Directions:

1. Put water in a pot, add some salt and bring to a boil over medium high heat.
2. Add green beans, cook for 5 minutes and transfer them to a bowl filled with ice water.
3. Drain green beans well and put them in a salad bowl.

4. Add walnuts, fennel and goat cheese and toss gently.
5. In a bowl, mix vinegar with mustard, salt, pepper and oil and whisk well.
6. Pour this over salad, toss to coat well and serve for lunch.

Enjoy!

Nutrition: calories 200, fat 14, fiber 4, carbs 5, protein 6

Pumpkin Soup

This keto soup is very creamy and textured! You should really try it for lunch today!

Preparation time: 10 minutes

Cooking time: 20 minutes

Servings: 6

Ingredients:

- ½ cup yellow onion, chopped
- 2 tablespoons olive oil
- 1 tablespoon chipotles in adobo sauce
- 1 garlic clove, minced
- 1 teaspoon cumin, ground
- 1 teaspoon coriander, ground
- A pinch of allspice
- 2 cups pumpkin puree
- Salt and black pepper to the taste
- 32 ounces chicken stock
- ½ cup heavy cream
- 2 teaspoons vinegar
- 2 teaspoons stevia

Directions:

1. Heat up a pot with the oil over medium heat, add onions and garlic, stir and cook for 4 minutes.
2. Add stevia, cumin, coriander, chipotles and cumin, stir and cook for 2 minutes.
3. Add stock and pumpkin puree, stir and cook for 5 minutes.
4. Blend soup well using an immersion blender and then mix with salt, pepper, heavy cream and vinegar.
5. Stir, cook for 5 minutes more and divide into bowls.
6. Serve right away.

Enjoy!

Nutrition: calories 140, fat 12, fiber 3, carbs 6, protein 2

Delicious Green Beans Casserole

This will impress you for sure!

Preparation time: 10 minutes

Cooking time: 35 minutes

Servings: 8

Ingredients:

- 1 pound green beans, halved
- Salt and black pepper to the taste
- ½ cup almond flour
- 2 tablespoons ghee
- 8 ounces mushrooms, chopped
- 4 ounces onion, chopped
- 2 shallots, chopped
- 3 garlic cloves, minced
- ½ cup chicken stock
- ½ cup heavy cream
- ¼ cup parmesan, grated
- Avocado oil for frying

Directions:

1. Put some water in a pot, add salt, bring to a boil over medium high heat, add green beans, cook for 5 minutes, transfer to a bowl filled with ice water, cool down, drain well and leave aside for now.
2. In a bowl, mix shallots with onions, almond flour, salt and pepper and toss to coat.
3. Heat up a pan with some avocado oil over medium high heat, add onions and shallots mix, fry until they are golden.
4. Transfer to paper towels and drain grease.
5. Heat up the same pan over medium heat, add ghee and melt it.
6. Add garlic and mushrooms, stir and cook for 5 minutes.
7. Add stock and heavy cream, stir, bring to a boil and simmer until it thickens.
8. Add parmesan and green beans, toss to coat and take off heat.
9. Transfer this mix to a baking dish, sprinkle crispy onions mix all over, introduce in the oven at 400 degrees F and bake for 15 minutes.
10. Serve warm.

Enjoy!

Nutrition: calories 155, fat, 11, fiber 6, carbs 8, protein 5

Simple Lunch Apple Salad

This is not just Ketogenic! It's also very tasty!

Preparation time: 10 minutes

Cooking time: 0 minutes

Servings: 4

Ingredients:

- 2 cups broccoli florets, roughly chopped
- 2 ounces pecans, chopped
- 1 apple, cored and grated
- 1 green onion stalk, finely chopped
- Salt and black pepper to the taste
- 2 teaspoons poppy seeds
- 1 teaspoon apple cider vinegar
- ¼ cup mayonnaise
- ½ teaspoon lemon juice
- ¼ cup sour cream

Directions:

1. In a salad bowl, mix apple with broccoli, green onion and pecans and stir.
2. Add poppy seeds, salt and pepper and toss gently.

3. In a bowl, mix mayo with sour cream, vinegar and lemon juice and whisk well.
4. Pour this over salad, toss to coat well and serve cold for lunch!

Enjoy!

Nutrition: calories 250, fat 23, fiber 4, carbs 4, protein 5

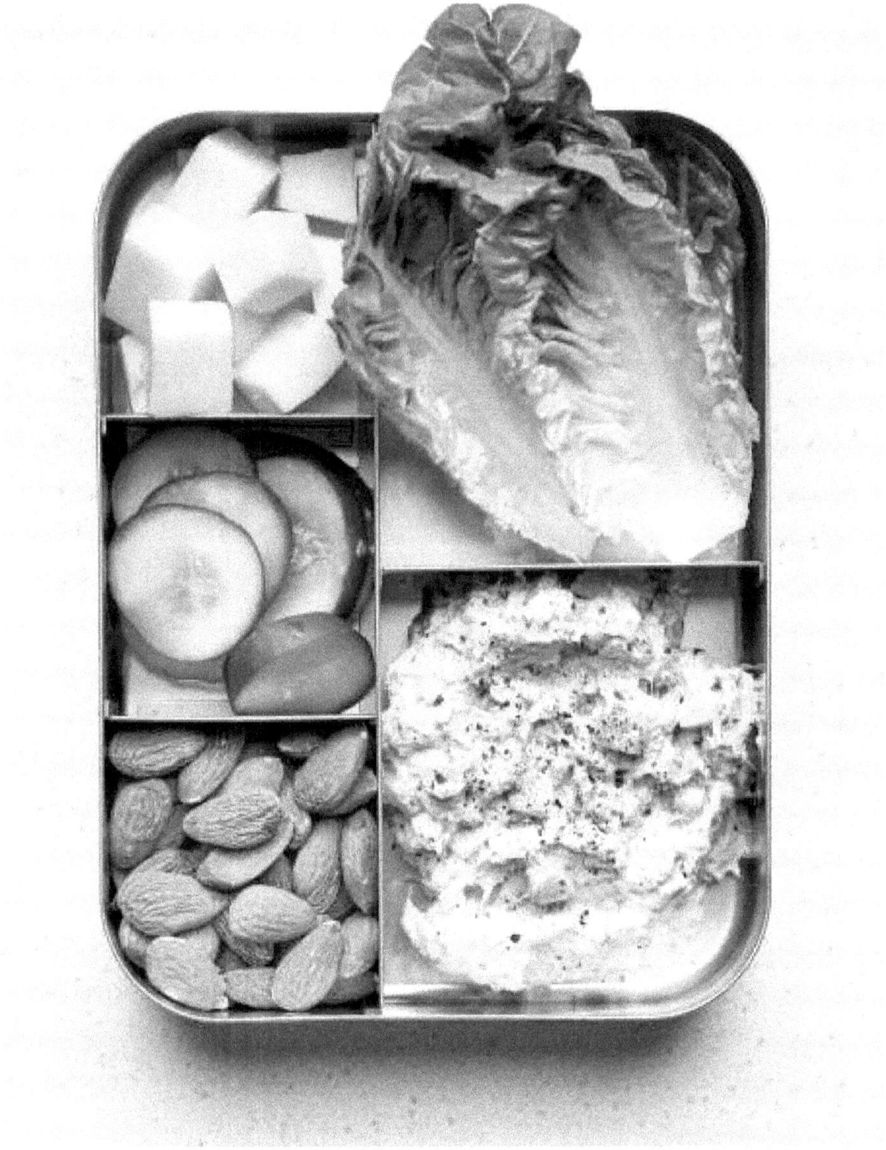

Brussels Sprouts Gratin

It's a dense and rich keto lunch idea!

Preparation time: 10 minutes

Cooking time: 35 minutes

Servings: 4

Ingredients:

- 2 ounces onions, chopped
- 1 teaspoon garlic, minced
- 6 ounces Brussels sprouts, chopped
- 2 tablespoons ghee
- 1 tablespoon coconut aminos
- Salt and black pepper to the taste
- ½ teaspoon liquid smoke

For the sauce:

- 2.5 ounces cheddar cheese, grated
- A pinch of black pepper
- 1 tablespoon ghee
- ½ cup heavy cream
- ¼ teaspoon turmeric
- ¼ teaspoon paprika
- A pinch of xanthan gum

For the pork crust:

- 3 tablespoons parmesan
- 0.5 ounces pork rinds
- ½ teaspoon sweet paprika

Directions:

1. Heat up a pan with 2 tablespoons ghee over high heat, add Brussels sprouts, salt and pepper, stir and cook for 3 minutes.
2. Add garlic and onion, stir and cook for 3 minutes more.
3. Add liquid smoke and coconut aminos, stir, take off heat and leave aside for now.
4. Heat up another pan with 1 tablespoon ghee over medium heat, add heavy cream and stir.
5. Add cheese, black pepper, turmeric, paprika and xanthan gum, stir and cook until it thickens again.
6. Add Brussels sprouts mix, toss to coat and divide into ramekins.
7. In your food processor, mix parmesan with pork rinds and ½ teaspoon paprika and pulse well.
8. Divide these crumbs on top of Brussels sprouts mix, introduce ramekins in the oven at 375 degrees F and bake for 20 minutes.
9. Serve right away.

Enjoy!

Nutrition: calories 300, fat 20, fiber 6, carbs 5, protein 10

Simple Asparagus Lunch

You only need a few ingredients and a few minutes of your time to make this simple and very tasty keto lunch!

Preparation time: 10 minutes

Cooking time: 10 minutes

Servings: 4

Ingredients:

- 2 egg yolks
- Salt and black pepper to the taste
- ¼ cup ghee
- 1 tablespoon lemon juice
- A pinch of cayenne pepper
- 40 asparagus spears

Directions:

1. In a bowl, whisk egg yolks very well.
2. Transfer this to a small pan over low heat.
3. Add lemon juice and whisk well.
4. Add ghee and whisk until it melts.
5. Add salt, pepper and cayenne pepper and whisk again well.

6. Meanwhile, heat up a pan over medium high heat, add asparagus spears and fry them for 5 minutes.
7. Divide asparagus on plates, drizzle the sauce you've made on top and serve.

Enjoy!

Nutrition: calories 150, fat 13, fiber 6, carbs 2, protein 3

Simple Shrimp Pasta

This is so yummy!

Preparation time: 10 minutes

Cooking time: 10 minutes

Servings: 4

Ingredients:

- 12 ounces angel hair noodles
- 2 tablespoons olive oil
- Salt and black pepper to the taste
- 2 tablespoons ghee
- 4 garlic cloves, minced
- 1 pound shrimp, raw, peeled and deveined
- Juice of ½ lemon
- ½ teaspoon paprika
- A handful basil, chopped

Directions:

1. Put water in a pot, add some salt, bring to a boil, add noodles, cook for 2 minutes, drain them and transfer to a heated pan.

2. Toast noodles for a few seconds, take off heat and leave them aside.
3. Heat up a pan with the ghee and olive oil over medium heat, add garlic, stir and brown for 1 minute.
4. Add shrimp and lemon juice and cook for 3 minutes on each side.
5. Add noodles, salt, pepper and paprika, stir, divide into bowls and serve with chopped basil on top.

Enjoy!

Nutrition: calories 300, fat 20, fiber 6, carbs 3, protein 30

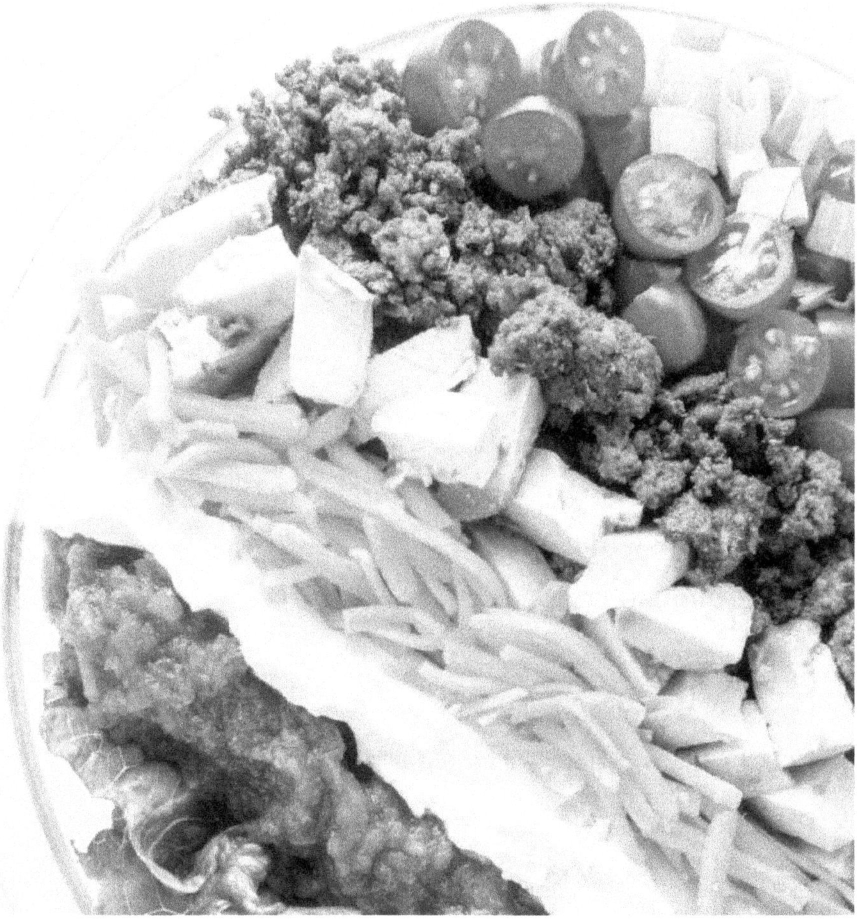

Cheese Tots

Prep time: 12 minutes

Cooking time: **3 minutes**

Servings: **5**

Ingredients:

- 8 oz. mozzarella balls
- 1 egg
- ½ cup coconut flakes
- ½ cup almond flour
- 1 teaspoon thyme
- 1 teaspoon ground black pepper
- 1 teaspoon paprika

Directions:

1. Beat the egg in the bowl and whisk it.
2. After this, combine the coconut flour with the thyme, ground black pepper, and paprika. Stir it carefully.
3. Then sprinkle Mozzarella balls with the coconut flakes.
4. After this, transfer the balls to the whisked egg mixture.
5. Then coat them in the almond flour mixture.
6. Put Mozzarella balls in the freezer for 5 minutes.
7. Meanwhile, preheat the air fryer to 400 F.

8. Put the frozen cheese balls in the preheated air fryer and cook them for 3 minutes.
9. When the time is over – remove the cheese tots from the air fryer basket and chill them for 2 minutes.
10. Serve the dish!

Nutrition: calories 166, fat 12.8, fiber 1.4, carbs 2.8, protein 9.5

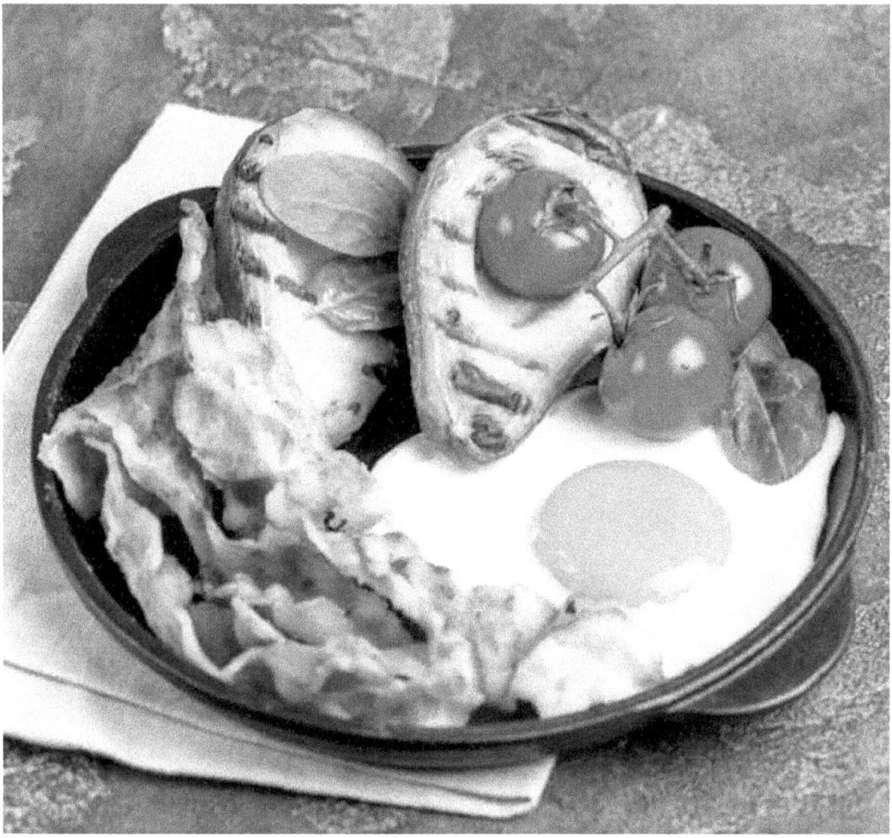

Sausage Balls

Prep time: 10 minutes

Cooking time: **8 minutes**

Servings: **5**

Ingredients:

- 8 oz. ground chicken
- 1 egg white
- 1 tablespoon dried parsley
- ½ teaspoon salt
- ½ teaspoon ground black pepper
- 2 tablespoon almond flour
- 1 tablespoon olive oil
- 1 teaspoon paprika
-

Directions:

1. Whisk the egg white and combine it with the ground chicken.
2. Sprinkle the chicken mixture with the dried parsley and salt.
3. After this, add the ground black pepper and paprika.
4. Stir the mass carefully using the spoon.

5. Then make the hands wet and make the small balls from the ground chicken mixture.
6. Sprinkle every sausage ball with the almond flour.
7. Preheat the air fryer to 380 F.
8. Then spray the air fryer basket tray with the olive oil inside and put the sausage balls there.
9. Cook the dish for 8 minutes.
10. You can turn the balls into another side during the cooking to get the brown color of the each side.
11. Transfer the cooked sausage balls in the serving plates.
12. Enjoy!

Nutrition: calories 180, fat 11.8, fiber 1.5, carbs 2.9, protein 16.3

Tofu Scramble

Prep time: 15 minutes

Cooking time: **20 minutes**

Servings: **5**

Ingredients:

- 10 oz tofu cheese
- 2 eggs
- 1 teaspoon chives
- 1 tablespoon apple cider vinegar
- ½ teaspoon salt
- 1 teaspoon ground white pepper
- ¼ teaspoon ground coriander

Directions:

1. Shred tofu cheese and sprinkle it with the apple cider vinegar, salt, ground white pepper, and ground coriander.
2. Mix it up and leave for 10 minutes to marinate.
3. Meanwhile, preheat the air fryer to 370 F.
4. Then transfer the marinated shredded tofu cheese in the air fryer basket tray and cook the cheese for 13 minutes.
5. Meanwhile, beat the eggs in the bowl and whisk them.

6. When the time is over – pour the egg mixture in the shredded tofu cheese and stir it with the help of the spatula well.
7. When the eggs start to be firm – place the air fryer basket tray in the air fryer and cook the dish for 7 minutes more.
8. After this, remove the cooked meal from the air fryer basket tray and serve it.
9. Enjoy!

Nutrition: calories 109, fat 6.7, fiber 1.4, carbs 2.9, protein 11.2

Hemp Seeds Porridge

Prep time: 10 minutes

Cooking time: **15 minutes**

Servings: **3**

Ingredients:

- 2 tablespoon flax seeds
- 4 tablespoon hemp seeds
- 1 tablespoon butter
- ¼ teaspoon salt
- 1 teaspoon stevia
- 7 tablespoon almond milk
- ½ teaspoon ground ginger

Directions:

1. Place the flax seeds and hemp seeds in the air fryer basket.
2. Sprinkle the seeds with the salt and ground ginger.
3. Combine the almond milk and stevia together. Stir the liquid and pour it in the seeds mixture.
4. After this, add butter.
5. Preheat the air fryer to 370 F and cook the hemp seeds porridge for 15 minutes.
6. Stir it carefully after 10 minutes of cooking.

7. When the time is over – remove the hem porridge from the air fryer basket tray and chill it for 3 minutes.
8. Transfer the Hemp Seeds porridge in the serving bowls.
9. Enjoy!

Nutrition: calories 196, fat 18.2, fiber 2.4, carbs 4.2, protein 5.1

Bacon Scrambled Eggs

Prep time: 10 minutes

Cooking time: **10 minutes**

Servings: **4**

Ingredients:

- 6 oz. bacon
- 4 eggs
- 5 tablespoon heavy cream
- 1 tablespoon butter
- 1 teaspoon paprika
- ½ teaspoon nutmeg
- 1 teaspoon salt
- 1 teaspoon ground black pepper

Directions:

1. Chop the bacon into the small pieces and sprinkle it with salt.
2. Stir the bacon gently and put in the air fryer basket.
3. Cook the chopped bacon in the preheated to 360 F air fryer for 5 minutes.
4. Meanwhile, beat the eggs in the bowl and whisk them using the hand whisker.

5. Sprinkle the whisked egg mixture with the paprika, nutmeg, and ground black pepper.
6. Whisk egg mixture gently again.
7. When the time is over – toss the butter in the chopped bacon and pour the egg mixture.
8. Add the heavy cream and cook it for 2 minutes.
9. After this, stir the mixture with the help of the spatula until you get the scrambled eggs and cook the dish for 3 minutes more.
10. Then transfer the cooked bacon scrambled eggs in the serving plates.
11. Enjoy!

Nutrition: calories 387, fat 32.1, fiber 0.4, carbs 2.3, protein 21.9

Delightful Breakfast Hash

Prep time: 8 minutes

Cooking time: **8 minutes**

Servings: **4**

Ingredients:

- 1 zucchini
- 7 oz. bacon, cooked
- 4 oz. Cheddar cheese
- 2 tablespoon butter
- 1 teaspoon salt
- 1 teaspoon ground black pepper
- 1 teaspoon paprika
- 1 teaspoon cilantro
- 1 teaspoon ground thyme

Directions:

1. Chop the zucchini into the small cubes and sprinkle it with the salt, ground black pepper, paprika, cilantro, and ground thyme.
2. Preheat the air fryer to 400 F and toss the butter in the air fryer basket tray.
3. Melt it and add the zucchini cubes.
4. Cook the zucchini for 5 minutes.

5. Meanwhile, shred Cheddar cheese.
6. When the time is over – shake the zucchini cubes carefully and add the cooked bacon.
7. Sprinkle the zucchini mixture with the shredded cheese and cook it for 3 minutes more.
8. When the time is over – transfer the breakfast hash in the serving bowls and stir.
9. Enjoy!

Nutrition: calories 445, fat 36.1, fiber 1, carbs 3.5, protein 26.3

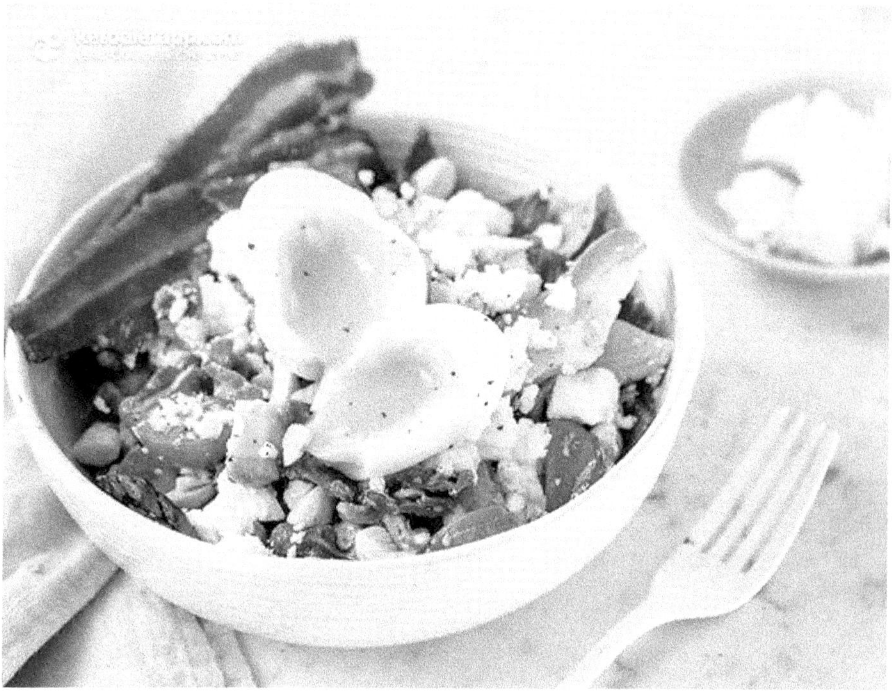

Cheddar Soufflé with Greens

Prep time: 10 minutes

Cooking time: **8 minutes**

Servings: **4**

Ingredients:

- 5 oz. Cheddar cheese, shredded
- 3 eggs
- 4 tablespoon heavy cream
- 1 tablespoon chives
- 1 tablespoon dill
- 1 teaspoon parsley
- ½ teaspoon ground thyme

Directions:

1. Crack the eggs into the bowl and whisk them carefully.
2. After this, add the heavy cream and whisk it for 10 seconds more.
3. Then add the chives, dill, parsley, and ground thyme.
4. Sprinkle the egg mixture with the shredded cheese and stir it.
5. Transfer the egg mixture in 4 ramekins and put the ramekins in the air fryer basket.

6. Preheat the air fryer to 390 F and cook the soufflé for 8 minutes.
7. When the time is over and the soufflé is cooked – chill it well.
8. Enjoy!

Nutrition: calories 244, fat 20.6, fiber 0.2, carbs 1.7, protein 13.5

Bacon Biscuits

Prep time: 15 minutes

Cooking time: **10 minutes**

Servings: **6**

Ingredients:

- 1 egg
- 4 oz. bacon, cooked
- 1 cup almond flour
- ½ teaspoon baking soda
- 1 tablespoon apple cider vinegar
- 3 tablespoon butter
- 4 tablespoon heavy cream
- 1 teaspoon dried oregano

Directions:

1. Beat the egg in the bowl and whisk it.
2. Chop the cooked bacon into the small cubes and add it in the whisked egg.
3. Then sprinkle the mixture with the baking soda and apple cider vinegar.
4. Add the heavy cream and dried oregano. Stir it.
5. After this, add butter and almond flour.
6. Mix it up with the help of the hand mixer.

7. When you get the smooth and liquid batter – the dough is cooked.
8. Preheat the air fryer to 400 F.
9. Pour the batter dough into the muffin molds.
10. When the air fryer is preheated – put the muffin forms in the air fryer basket and cook them for 10 minutes.
11. When the time is over and the muffins are prepared – remove them from the air fryer.
12. Chill the muffins till the room temperature.
13. Serve!

Nutrition: calories 226, fat 20.5, fiber 0.6, carbs 1.8, protein 9.2

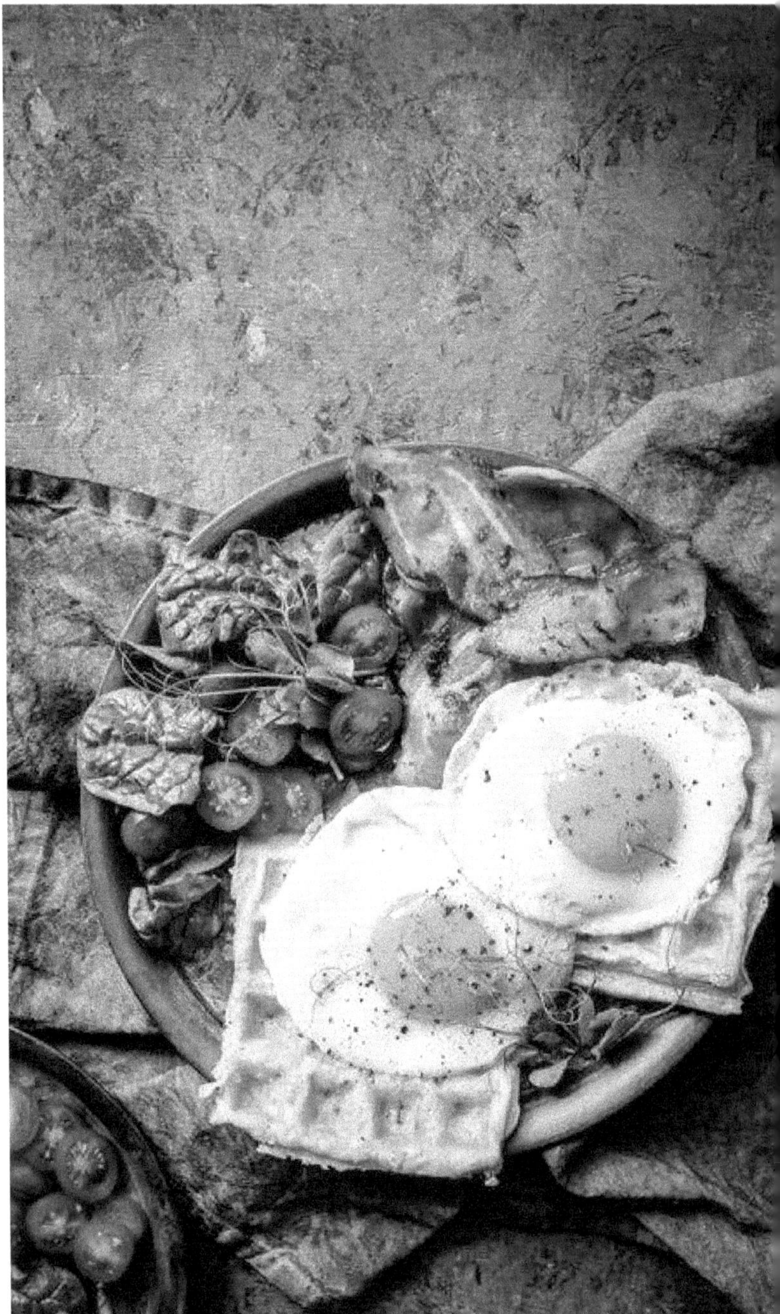

Keto Frittata

Prep time: 10 minutes

Cooking time: **15 minutes**

Servings: **6**

Ingredients:

- 6 eggs
- 1/3 cup heavy cream
- 1 tomato
- 1/2 onion
- 1 tablespoon butter
- 1 teaspoon salt
- 1 tablespoon dried oregano
- 6 oz. Parmesan
- 1 teaspoon chili pepper

Directions:

1. Beat the eggs in the air fryer basket tray and whisk them with the help of the hand whisker.
2. After this, chop the tomato and dice the onion.
3. Add the vegetables to the egg mixture.
4. Then pour the heavy cream.
5. Sprinkle the liquid mixture with the butter, salt, dried oregano, and chili pepper.

6. Then shred Parmesan cheese and add it to the mixture too.
7. Sprinkle the mixture with the silicone spatula.
8. Preheat the air fryer to 375 F and cook the frittata for 15 minutes.
9. When the time is over – transfer frittata in the serving plates.
10. Enjoy!

Nutrition: calories 202, fat 15, fiber 0.7, carbs 3.4, protein 15.1

16.1

Milton Keynes UK
Ingram Content Group UK Ltd.
UKHW022304020124
435363UK00015B/1426